Coconut Oil Ha

Nature's Miracle for Weight Loss, Hair Loss, and a Beautiful You!

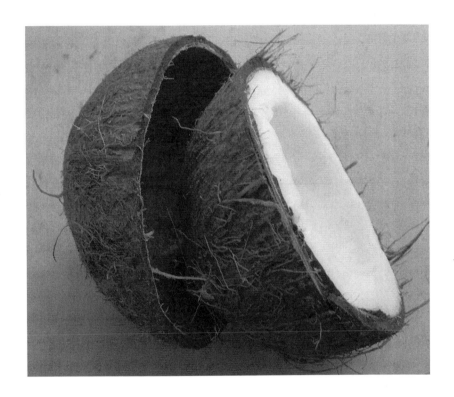

By Joshua Collins

Copyright

Coconut Oil Handbook: Nature's Miracle for Weight Loss, Hair Loss and a Beautiful You!

© Copyright 2013 Joshua Collins

First Published, 2013

Printed in the United States of America

Table of Contents

Coconut Oil: Natures Miracle for Weight Loss, Hair Loss and a Beautiful You!

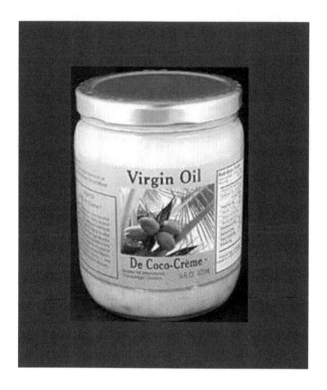

For many years the media and the majority of health care professionals have been telling us that saturated fats are bad for your health. Saturated fats, we have been told will lead us down the path to poor health. These types of fats have been blamed for conditions like elevated cholesterol, heart disease, obesity, Alzheimer's disease and many other abnormal degenerative conditions in our bodies.

In the meantime if you look at the statistics, for example, of heart disease and other degenerative conditions and you will also notice a drastic increase in these maladies in recent years in spite of the abundance of low saturated fat diets and literature available to the public on the negative effects of saturated fats. Did you know that there have been multiple studies conducted on Pacific Island populations who ingest saturated Coconut Oil on a daily basis? What is interesting is that coconut oil accounts for up to 30-60% of their daily caloric intake. These same studies have shown that the incidence of cardiovascular disease is almost non-existent in these populations.

Clearly, there is a lot of confusion in relation to the subject of saturated fats, and this confusion even exists among health care professionals today. The chemistry of saturated fats is very complicated and my goal is not to give you a chemistry lesson but rather to educate you about the positive benefits of Coconut Oil.

The moral of the story is that not all saturated fats are created equal and in fact the naturally occurring saturated fats like coconut oil are in fact beneficial to our health in many ways.

Coconut Oil in its unrefined state consists of 92% saturated fatty acids, 6% of mono-unsaturated fatty acids, and 2% of polyunsaturated fatty acids.

Saturated Fatty Acids Found in Coconut Oil

Saturated Fat is made up of triglycerides that only contain saturated fatty acids. The main fatty acids found in Coconut Oil are Lauric Acid, Caprylic Acid, Palmitic Acid, Capric Acid, and Myristic Acid.

It is estimated that lauric acid, a fatty acid, makes up approximately 50% of coconut oil. It is this high concentration of lauric acid that has been theorized to provide the numerous health benefits of coconut oil. Lauric acid gets converted into monolaurin in our bodies. Monolaurin has been known to have antibacterial, anti-viral and antiprotozoal properties.

The saturated fats which are prevalent in coconut oil are a source of fuel for the body. They aid in absorption of vitamins that are fat-soluble, and they also assist in the absorption of phytonutrients, which are used in the body to build cell membranes.

Medium Chain Fatty Acids – The Miracle Molecules in Coconut Oil

Most of the fats we consume in our daily diets are of the long chain fatty acid variety. Being long chain they must be broken down before they can be absorbed. Coconut Oil is nature's richest source of short and medium chain fatty acids.

The beauty of these molecules is that they are easily digested and absorbed and are sent directly to the liver for energy production.

Medium chain fatty acids, also known as MCFA, are fats composed of capric and caprylic acids. What makes them unique is that they tend to resemble and behave more like carbohydrates than they do fats.

Unlike traditional fats they tend to be more water soluble. They do not require bile to break them down, and they also are broken down more quickly than long chain fats. They enter the blood stream quickly and are taken directly to the liver. Medium chain fatty acids provide a quick source of energy as well, however, since they are not a carbohydrate they do not stimulate insulin secretion. Because they are not dependent on insulin to be metabolized and broken down there is less likelihood of fat storage and that is where the weight reducing properties come into play.

MCFAs also stimulate thermogenesis whereby the body burns fat and produces heat. This is a good thing for people who are trying to lose weight.

Coconut Oil consists of about 66% medium chain fatty acids. These types of fatty acids are responsible for the tremendous amount of health benefits including but not limited to thyroid stimulation, weight loss, accelerated healing and an increase in the metabolic rate.

How can Coconut Oil Benefit your Health

Coconut Oil, in addition to the medium chain fatty acids, is rich in Vitamin E, Vitamin K and Iron. It also contains compounds such as phenolic anti-oxidants that are known to help our systems in combating different kinds of health issues.

Boost Immunity

Lauric acid, capric acid, and caprylic acid, found in high concentrations in coconut oil, are lipid substances that possess antifungal, antibacterial, and antiviral properties. The Caprylic Acid found in Coconut Oil targets harmful bacteria and it is commonly used to help diminish excess candida (fungus or yeast) in our body. Coconut Oil is known to help strengthen your body's immune system.

Improve Digestion

Because the fatty acids in coconut oil are sent directly to the liver for digestion no bile or pancreatic enzymes are needed for digestion. The MCFA molecules are smaller than the long chain variety and they require less energy and fewer enzymes to break them down for digestion. They tend to be digested quickly and absorbed with minimal effort. This makes coconut oil a healthy food even for those with diabetes or those who have gallbladder problems.

Researchers have demonstrated the benefits of Coconut Oil in patients with many different types of digestive problems. People suffering with Ulcerative Colitis Crohn's disease and other types of inflammatory bowel diseases have benefited from the ingestion of Coconut Oil. It is the anti-inflammatory and healing effects of coconut oil in addition to its easy digestibility, that play a role in soothing inflammation in the digestive tract which are characteristic of these inflammatory digestive diseases.

Stimulate Healing of Wounds and Infections

Pure Coconut Oil can also be used to heal wounds and scarring caused by infections. One of the key components of this oil is lauric acid, which has been proven scientifically to facilitate the healing process in addition to having anti-microbial properties.

Improve Your Thyroid Function With Coconut Oil

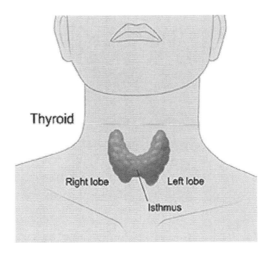

Approximately 27 million Americans are suffering from thyroid related diseases. Coconut Oil is an affordable way to keep your thyroid healthy. Coconut Oil stimulates your thyroid which can help maintain your metabolism's natural rhythm. This occurs because the medium chain fatty acids present in Coconut Oil have the properties of raising your metabolic rate and basal body temperature which will promote weight loss and increase your energy. These basic functions of the body are altered when your thyroid gland is not functioning properly.

Coconut Oil Promotes Healthy Cholesterol Levels

Coconut Oil helps lower cholesterol. It contains high concentration of Lauric Acid which guards our heart from the bad type of cholesterol (LDL). Coconut Oil also helps increase good cholesterol (HDL) to keep your heart and vascular system healthy and strong. If you study the literature on different types of oils you will see that it is the unsaturated oils that have been implicated in heart disease. We will be discussing cholesterol later in more detail because it is so important.

Coconut Oil and Blood Sugar Regulation

Coconut Oil aids in controlling blood sugar in our body because it does not produce a spike in the secretion of insulin when ingested as a food. Simple carbohydrates are touted as a quick source of energy for our bodies however they produce a rapid rise in insulin secretion which can literally bounce your blood sugars up and down very quickly which is unhealthy. Coconut Oil, on the other hand, is also a powerful source of instant energy for your body without the rapid rise and fall of your blood sugar levels. This is why it is effective in the stabilization of blood sugars in diabetics.

Coconut Oil and Cardiovascular Health

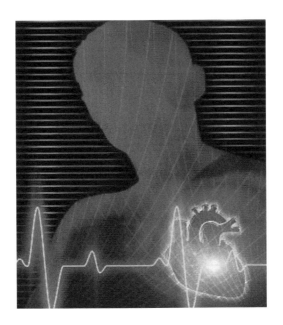

Coconut Oil helps reduce the risk of heart disease. Because it is stable in cooking when it is heated it does not form free radicals which have been implicated in the cause of degenerative diseases such as heart disease. Polyunsaturated fats present in vegetable oils and seed oils tend to encourage the formation of blood clots. This is because these polyunsaturated oils increase the stickiness of platelets which are responsible for clotting in our bodies. Coconut Oil helps to promote normal platelet function and thereby reduces platelet stickiness.

The cholesterol modulating effect of Coconut oil which we have previously discussed as well as the weight loss function also contributes to your cardiovascular health.

Non-Medicinal uses for Coconut Oil

Coconut Oil is a multi-purpose substance that is admired by many because it is effective, safe and has many uses that you may not be aware of. You probably have heard that Coconut Oil is good for skin care and hair care. What you will come to understand is that Coconut Oil has a lot more to offer and has many other uses.

Coconut Oil for Shaving

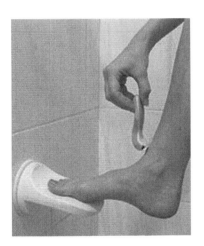

After shaving, it is pretty common for our skin to feel a little irritated and possibly itchy. Sometimes, the chemical laden shaving gels and creams we use may cause this irritation to our skin. It is hard to think of any better shaving moisturizer than Coconut Oil. So if you use it for shaving it will not cause the skin to become irritated. It will leave your face if you are a man and your legs if you are a woman silky smooth. In fact the coconut oil will leave your skin clean, soft and deeply moisturized.

Coconut Oil for Brushing Teeth

Because of Coconut Oils antibacterial properties, it can be used as an effectively as your regular toothpaste. All you have to do is simply make your own homemade toothpaste by mixing Coconut Oil and baking soda. Just mix 2 tablespoons of pure coconut oil with 2 tablespoons of high quality baking soda, and then add 10 drops of peppermint to add flavor and you will have a great tasting, cavity fighting and plaque reducing toothpaste.

Coconut Oil for Oil Pulling Therapy

For those of you who have never heard of it, Oil Pulling Therapy is an ancient native Indian folk remedy. It is simply done by swishing Coconut Oil in your mouth. It is an effective way to fight off oral problems such as gingivitis, halitosis and oral plaque. Coconut Oil can be used effectively for oil pulling therapy because of its antibacterial properties.

Coconut Oil for as a Natural Deodorant

Coconut Oil can be used as an effective deodorant. If you are one of those individuals that sweat excessively which tends to produce an odor you can replace your chemical-based deodorant with an all-natural Coconut Oil. It is more economical, safe and absolutely a match from heaven for sensitive skin. You will also love the aroma of coconut oil as a natural deodorizer.

Coconut Oil for Removing Make-Up

Oh how women love putting on make-up and how they hate the process of removing it. It is time consuming and usually leaves ones facial skin irritated and red especially when it is not done properly. If you rub your skin with soap and water to remove makeup, the oils your skin naturally secretes and any residues from the day, you can damage your facial skin. If you want an absolutely better and cheaper way to remove make-up, you have to make use of Coconut Oil.

Using Coconut Oil to clean your face is very simple. Warm an ample amount of Coconut Oil between your palm or finger tips. Then, massage your face with it. You will immediately notice that your make-up loosens and becomes very easy to remove with no vigorous rubbing required. Simply wet a clean and soft washcloth with warm water and delicately massage away any make-up residues on your face. Repeat the process if necessary.

Coconut Oil for all Your Hair Care Needs

Coconut Oil is useful for practically every hair type. It helps to keep your hair shiny, soft, dandruff-free and damage-free. Coconut Oil works by reducing the loss of your hair's natural proteins in both damaged and undamaged hair. Because of the fact that it is 100% natural, Coconut Oil is considered to be better than any artificial or man-made hair treatments found in the market. Coconut Oil does not contain harmful chemicals, silicones and alcohols that may irritate the skin and scalp.

Coconut Oil has compounds that are known to promote healthy, shiny and thicker strands of hair. Coconut Oil acts as a conditioner and is scientifically proven to protect hair from getting damaged from a phenomenon called Hygral Fatigue. Essentially what happens with this type of fatigue is that when hair is wet, it absorbs water and swells. As it dries, especially if you are using a hair dryer, it releases water and shrivels. This frequent shrinking and swelling can lead to damaged hair follicles. A good analogy is when you continually stretch a rubber band eventually it loses its elasticity and becomes limp. This is exactly what happens to hair.

Condition your Hair with Coconut Oil

You can treat damaged and frizzy hair caused by heat styling, dyeing, bleaching, perming, straightening and other chemical treatments. Coconut Oil will be your godsend solution. It is not only safe to use, it is also easy to apply. All you have to do is massage at least 3 tablespoons of Coconut Oil onto your hair and scalp and leave it for a good 20-30 minutes to make sure that penetrates hair and scalp deeply.

You can wrap your hair with a hot towel or simply cover it with a shower cap to enhance the Coconut Oil's effect on your hair and scalp. You will need to shampoo your hair after the treatment because Coconut Oil can make your hair feel heavy and greasy. Be sure to a use mild and damage reducing shampoos to remove the Coconut Oil after a treatment.

Coconut Oil for Moisturizing your Scalp and Treating Dandruff

You can use Coconut Oil to get rid of that nasty dandruff problem. Dandruff is usually caused by a dry scalp. The lack of moisture is what makes it flaky. Since Coconut Oil is a great moisturizer, a small amount massaged into the scalp for ten or more minutes can help you finally say goodbye to dandruff. It is best if you choose to use 100% pure Virgin Coconut Oil for best results. This remedy, unlike other medical treatments or home remedies for dandruff is100% safe. There will be no stinging, no itching, and definitely no pain associated with its use. If you treat your hair with Coconut Oil, your scalp can be dandruff free for up to 6 months.

Coconut Oil for Getting Rid of Head Lice

I know you probably think head lice infestation is due to unsanitary conditions in one's home and that couldn't happen to you or your child. If you think it is not possible just just call your local nurse at your local elementary school and you will find out it is very common problem in young children and highly contagious. Head Lice are very tiny parasitic wingless insects that lay eggs on the hair strands. Head lice infestation is literally one irritating problem to have. It not only makes your hair itchy, it can also make your hair and scalp unhealthy. If you want to have an effective natural solution for this nasty hair problem, Coconut Oil may be your answer.

Coconut Oil is safe to use and both children and adults can use for this kind of treatment. Coconut Oil can and will kill head lice. What it does is it makes the tiny insects die from dehydration. All you have to do is apply Coconut oil from your scalp to the tip of your hair and then cover your head with a plastic shower cap. Leave it for 5 to 6 hours to maximize its effects (better to do it overnight). Clean your hair with mild shampoo and your head will be lice free for good.

Understanding Hair Loss and How Coconut Oil Can Help

We have all heard about how great coconut oil is; it has been proven over the long run that it promotes great benefits to your health and wellness. But one thing that many are not fully aware of is how good this natural oil is for the hair and not just as a conditioner or a scalp cleanser. Let's face it; many people experience hair-related problems that are not just limited to a simple case of dandruff. Some have weak and brittle hair that breaks easily. Others have a bigger battle that often makes them feel like they're on the losing end – no pun intended; and that battle is against hair loss. Fortunately for all of us who suffer from this problem, coconut oil can help in a big way.

What's in Coconut Oil Anyway?

Just to refresh your memory Coconut oil has more to offer than just being a "good" healthy saturated fat. Apart from possessing Vitamin E, Vitamin K, and Iron that are all good for the hair repair and growth, it also contains a wide variety of fatty acids that serve as excellent emollients. These include the following:

• Linoleic Acid

- Capric Acid

- Oleic Acid

- Lauric Acid

- Palmitic Acid

- Myristic Acid

- Caprylic Acid

What's the Real Deal with Hair Loss?

There are many potential problems that affect – or promote hair loss. However, the root of the problem is often the matter of how healthy the hair and scalp is. If your hair or scalp is not maintained properly, there is always a chance of experiencing hair loss even if you are not genetically prone to acquire it.

Dry and Unhealthy Scalp – When your scalp does not have the necessary moisture that it needs, it will not be able to support your hair follicles, let alone your hair as it grows. Do note that moisture is not the only thing that matters; your scalp also needs nutrition. If your scalp is also riddled with skin conditions such as acne, dandruff, eczema, etc. this will also promote hair loss.

Dry Hair – Dry hair is a clear indication that it is not healthy. It means that your follicles are not receiving the proper nutrition they need to promote good hair growth. If this is the case, your hair will likely grow slowly and it will tend to break easily, split, and ultimately fall out.

Artificial Factors – This is often used to explain hair loss. It is attributed to hair that is frequently chemically-treated with either dyes, straightening agents, or with shampoos that contain harsh chemical (sulfates) ingredients. Hair can also become weakened and unhealthy when it is constantly subject to hair irons, curlers, and blow dryers due to the heat factor.

How Coconut Oil Can Help Hair Loss

Coconut oil, because of the nutritional content that is has, provides the ability to restore nutrition to your hair and scalp. Chemically treated and constantly styled hair tends to be stressed. Because it is also an excellent emollient it has the ability to restore moisture to your hair and leave it soft and silky smooth.

Coconut oil also has the ability to restore and promote protein growth in the hair. Protein loss is one of the most common reasons for hair loss. With the help of coconut oil, the hair shaft, cuticle, and every single hair strand will get the proper nourishment it needs to repair any damage that has occurred.

On another note, coconut oil has antifungal, antimicrobial, and antioxidant properties that also helps in averting hair loss. This means that if your scalp is suffering from any parasites, or medical condition that renders it unable to support and promote healthy hair growth, regular use of coconut oil can oftentimes cure it.

Many have claimed that this oil is a miracle solution to hair loss. The truth is there is no miracle in it. The key is simply the coconut oil's ability to restore proper moisture and nutrition to the hair and scalp that promotes strong and health hair. Experts will agree that experiencing hair loss is next to unlikely if its condition never falls short of health.

How to Use Coconut Oil to Promote Hair Growth

Coconut Oil comes in a solid form due to its high melting temperature but melts into a liquid state when in contact with heat. One thing I recommend is to never microwave this oil. Instead, place the jar in hot water until it turns to a liquid.

Dampen hair with warm water.

Spoon Coconut Oil from the jar into your hands and apply directly to your roots covering your scalp. Use two tablespoons of oil for shoulder length hair and three to four tablespoons for longer hair.

Massage the oil into your scalp for at least two to three minutes. It is possible that you may see hair fall from the massage, but do not fret–your scalp is adjusting to the stimulation. If it bothers you, skip this step.

If you desire, you may cover the length of your hair with the oil as well for an overall conditioning treatment.

Put your oiled hair in a shower cap to let the treatment set.

Leave the oil treatment on your hair for no less than 20 minutes. It is optimal if you leave it in overnight, but 20 minutes is enough for a treatment if you're short on time. Repeat this treatment two to three times per week for a minimum of three months.

After your desired length of treatment, wash the oil out with a sulfate free shampoo. You will not feel the need to condition your hair, as silky softness is an immediate benefit of this treatment.

After one to two weeks, you will see an improvement in your overall hair quality and possibly some new growth! Many who have used Coconut Oil treatments a minimum of three months and have had a number of inches of new growth on their scalps in that amount of time!

Coconut Oil and Skin Care

Coconut Oil is considered to be an all-in-one natural solution for all skin types. It is proven to be safe and effective to use from head to toe. It offers an all-in-one package for skin care. It has the right amount of nutrients and vitamins to keep our skin soft, smooth, younger looking and healthy. Coconut Oil is simply a complete skin care package – moisturizer, multivitamin, antibiotic, anti-aging and anti-oxidant.

One of the major benefits of Coconut Oil is that it helps increase the elasticity of the skin which is good news to all the wrinkle conscious people out there who are concerned about premature aging.

Coconut Oil is also used to treat skin problems such as dermatitis, psoriasis and eczema.

Coconut Oil as Skin Moisturizer

Coconut Oil is effective in helping to get rid of dry and flaky skin. Rub it on your skin to keep it hydrated throughout the day.

Coconut Oil as Skin Emollient

Since Coconut Oil is filled with natural and essential fatty acids, it works great at keeping your skin soft and smooth. You can get rid of dry and itchy skin by using Coconut Oil. It can also soften and help heal minor skin wounds faster.

Coconut Oil as a Skin Antioxidant

You will immediately fall in love with Coconut Oil knowing that it is an excellent antioxidant which helps prevent premature aging and wrinkling. You are living in a fast-paced world filled with environmental pollutants and unhealthy foods that can cause free radicals to build up in your body. These free radicals have the ability to damage your healthy cells.

To ward off these free radicals, you can commit to practice a healthy lifestyle which includes taking adequate amounts of antioxidants. Coconut Oil is a skin antioxidant that can keep your skin elastic and adaptable to bodily changes. Coconut oil can keep your skin smooth, healthy, and wrinkle free.

Coconut Oil is Food for the Skin

Coconut Oil can is considered food for the skin because of it contains nourishing nutrients and fatty acids. These nutrients and fatty acids can be easily absorbed by the skin and directly feeds the mitochondria of your cells which are the power houses of healthy living cells. These nutrients will provide the cells of your skin with energy to naturally recover and repair itself. Use Coconut Oil to keep your skin healthy and energized.

Coconut Oil as an Antibacterial for the Skin

The active fatty acids that Coconut Oil contains are Lauric Acid, Caprylic Acid and Capric Acid. These acids are clinically proven to provide safe antibacterial, antifungal, and antiviral effect on your skin. It is now being considered and tested as a form of treatment for the HIV virus. Yes, Coconut Oil is that powerful.

Coconut Oil as an Acne Buster

Coconut oil can be a powerful substance that helps get rid of acne. Its antibiotic properties can effectively eliminate the bacteria which cause acne. Coconut Oil can also be used to heal your acne scarring which results from a chronic infection of the skin.

Coconut Oil as a Skin Deodorizer

You can shower with Coconut Oil to keep your skin fresh and clean. It is a safe and natural way to deodorize your body. Coconut Oil is very cheap so you do not have to think twice about using it all over your body. Just ensure that you are purchasing unrefined pure virgin coconut oil to maximize the benefits.

Coconut Oil and Cholesterol

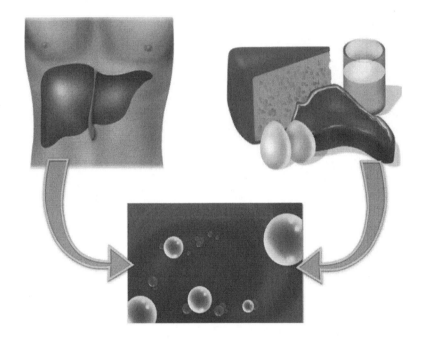

It is quite possible that you are thinking that Coconut Oil, because it is a saturated fat it will increase your cholesterol levels. In fact most of the literature on coconut oil and cholesterol levels is very misleading. By ingesting coconut oil you can keep your cholesterol at healthy values and can decrease your risk of heart disease. What actually happens is that coconut oil tends to increase what we call the good cholesterol known as HDL (high density lipoprotein).

So what is HDL Cholesterol?

Coconut Oil increases High Density Lipoprotein (HDL) component of cholesterol. The HDL cholesterol is considered by many as the good cholesterol because it is essential for normal body function. It is responsible for keeping every cell in your body healthy and stable by warding off low density lipoprotein (LDL) cholesterol, also known as the bad cholesterol.

HDL Cholesterol carries the LDL Cholesterol towards the liver for it to be reprocessed and reused. It is also responsible for keeping the endothelium (inner walls of blood vessels) clean and healthy. If there is lack of HDL Cholesterol and the endothelium gets destroyed, strokes and heart attacks can occur. Although Coconut Oil does not reduce Total Cholesterol, it keeps your Cholesterol Ratio at healthy levels.

The important Cholesterol Ratio

Having your doctor check your total cholesterol is not enough. In fact, it is quite misleading at times in checking your risk of heart disease. If you really want a more accurate test, ask your doctor for your Cholesterol Ratio instead. It will basically show you how much HDL Cholesterol you have in relation to LDL Cholesterol.

It is better from a health standpoint to have a low cholesterol ratio. If your cholesterol ratio is 5.0 milligrams per deciliter you have average risk of heart disease. The higher your cholesterol ratio the greater is your risk for heart disease. If your cholesterol ratio is 3.2 milligrams per deciliter or less, it means that you have a lower risk of heart disease. Furthermore, it is better to have your HDL Cholesterol at levels greater than 60 milligrams per deciliter to protect your heart.

If you need to increase your HDL Cholesterol, you can combine using Coconut Oil with these effective tips:

•Exercise – increase your HDL Cholesterol levels by using Coconut Oil and exercising for 30 minutes to an hour regularly.

•Stop Smoking – one of the many harmful effects of smoking is that it lowers your HDL Cholesterol levels. Quit smoking and keep using Coconut Oil to increase HDL cholesterol levels in your body.

•Avoid Obesity – keep a healthy weight to improve your HDL cholesterol levels. Obesity causes heart disease and other illnesses so ingest healthy Coconut Oil, eat healthy food, and have a healthy lifestyle.

Coconut Oil and Dieting

You might not think that Coconut Oil is good for dieting because of its high percentage of saturated fat, but that is where you are mistaken.

How Can Coconut Oil be used in Your Daily Diet?

Because the medium chained fatty acids found in Coconut Oil are less likely to be stored as fat in the body it has been used effectively for dieting. Medium chained saturated fats are also scientifically proven to speed up the fat burning process in our body which is called thermogenesis. That being said, Coconut Oil is a safe and effective way shed some pounds.

By taking one tablespoon of Coconut Oil 20 minutes before your meals every day, you will be enhancing your ability to lose weight. It will decrease your appetite and will make you feel full which in itself will curb your eating. The medium chained triglycerides in Coconut Oil will also increase your metabolism. It will also promote thermogenesis which will help you burn fat.

Coconut Oil has a nutty, subtle taste and can be used to enhance most recipes. You can replace your regular cooking oil with the much healthier Coconut Oil. You can incorporate Coconut Oil in your daily recipes to promote fat burning and easy digestion.

Coconut Oil can be used to make baked goods, desserts, beverages, soups, candies, spreads and other oil blends. These foods are healthy but if losing weight is what you really want to achieve, you know how you need to reduce the amount of calories you are ingesting and exercise. The moral of the story is you need to eat healthier foods, reduce your caloric intake and exercise so that you are burning more calories than you are ingesting and the weight will come off with perseverance and dedication.

What Type of Coconut Oil is good for me?

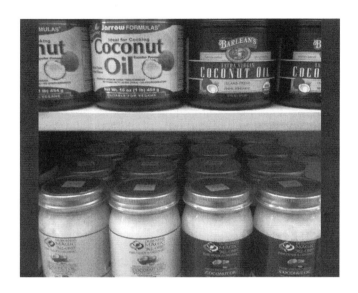

There are two major types of Coconut Oil. One is the mass produced refined Coconut Oil. When we say refined we mean that it is more likely that the coconuts used to make this type of coconut oil have been smoked or sun dried.

Since this type of drying process is somewhat unsanitary, the manufacturers will bleach, purify and deodorize the Coconut Oil they have extracted. This means that chemicals are used for the production of this kind of Coconut Oil and they remain in the oil when it is packaged. Therefore, it should be avoided and is not good for to consume.

What you should purchase is Pure Organic Virgin Coconut Oil. This type of Coconut Oil is extracted using sanitary and traditional methods which still leave its faint and distinct coconut taste.

If it is your first time purchasing pure organic virgin coconut oil, you should start with one small container or jar to experiment with. Then, as you get more and more accustomed to its taste, you can consider purchasing larger quantities online. If you do not like the taste of Coconut, you can purchase an expeller pressed coconut oil.

Coconut Oil and Weight Loss

In the past, Coconut Oil was considered unhealthy because of its high concentration of saturated fats. But recent studies have shown that Coconut Oil is beneficial for people who are trying to lose weight.

Before we go on to the details, let us first discuss how Coconut Oil's high concentration of saturated fats is harmless. The saturated fats that are found in Coconut Oil are very distinct. They are known as Medium Chain Triglycerides or MCTs. MCTs are unlike other saturated fats because they are metabolized very differently.

Contrary to saturated fats, MCTs are very rarely stored as body fat. MCTs are most likely to be converted to energy and therefore will not add weight to your body. According to one study made in the International Journal of Obesity and Metabolic Disorders, MCTs found in Coconuts or Coconut Oils can increase the fat burning and calorie expenditure process which will ultimately lead to a substantial reduction of fat storage.

How to Use Coconut Oil to Speed up your Weight Loss

Not all Coconut Oils are created the same, so before you use Coconut Oil to lose weight, make sure that you will only use pure organic virgin coconut oil. This will assure you that your Coconut Oil has not been processed by chemicals of any kind and it is safe to ingest.

Pure Organic Virgin Coconut Oil typically solidifies at 76 degrees Fahrenheit so it is advisable that you melt it in warm water before ingesting it.

Tips on Melting Pure Organic Virgin Coconut Oil

•Put one to two tablespoons of pure organic virgin coconut oil in a mug.

•Add hot water. You may also mix it with herbal tea if you prefer.

•Stir until it is in pure liquid form and drink.

When Should I Take Pure Organic Virgin Coconut Oil?

Take your dose of pure organic virgin coconut oil 20 minutes before having your meals. This should be done to significantly diminish your appetite. It will also make you feel full and satisfied shortly after consuming small portions of food.

You may also use Coconut Oil instead of regular cooking oil to cook your food. This way you reduce the amount of cholesterol and unhealthy saturated fats in your body. Replace the unhealthy oils you ingest with Coconut Oil and see amazing and visible weight loss results.

Tips on Cooking with Coconut Oil

You made the right decision when you chose to replace your regular cooking oil with Coconut Oil. It is definitely a lot healthier and it may even reduce your likelihood of gaining weight.

Now that you have decided to replace your vegetable oils in your kitchen with Coconut Oil there are a few things you should know. In most Asian countries this kind of oil is commonly used for cooking. If you haven't used coconut oil for cooking before, below are some tips on how you can incorporate it in your cooking.

Here are a few ideas on how Coconut Oil can be used in food Preparation

Jazz up your smoothies and Protein Shakes

You can add a twist of tropical flavor to your smoothie, protein shake, yogurt, fruit juice, apple sauce or cottage cheese and make them luscious by adding a spoonful of melted coconut oil in them.

Make your own Healthy Mayonnaise

Make healthy mayonnaise with the use of Coconut Oil. You just have to mix 2 egg yolks with 1 teaspoon of mustard. Add 1 teaspoon of balsamic vinegar and a little lemon juice. Add a pinch of pepper and salt. Then mix everything with 1 cup of pure organic virgin coconut oil.

Add Coconut Oil to your Salad Dressings

If you love salad, you would love your salad dressing mixed with coconut oil even better.

Sauté your Vegetables in Coconut Oil

Instead of using your regular cooking oil when sauté your vegetables in coconut oil to ensure that it is healthy and give them a unique taste.

Use Coconut Oil to Lubricate your Baking Tins

Instead of using butter or margarine, you can use coconut oil to lubricate your baking tins, bowls or pans. It will add a faint but special coconut flavor to your baked goods.

Cook you Fresh Fish with Coconut Oil

Transform an ordinary fish dish into a gourmet meal by cooking plain fish fillet using Coconut Oil. Simply add salt, pepper and garlic to enhance its flavor.

Eating Healthy with Coconut Oil Recipes

The use of Coconut Oil in the kitchen does not end with it simply being in the form of cooking oil for frying. Coconut Oil can be used for many other healthy recipes. It is a great to include coconut oil in soups, sweets, or in breakfast, lunch and dinner meals. Here are a few of my favorite recipes:

Tropical Coconut Banana Pancakes

Ingredients:

Coconut oil for cooking
¼ liter of coconut milk
2 eggs
½ teaspoon of almond extract
7 ounces of flour (a little more than ¾ cup)
3.5 ounces of grated coconut (little less than ½ cup)
1 tablespoon of sugar
2 teaspoons of baking powder
½ teaspoon of salt
1 banana: sliced and quartered

Procedure:

Pancakes are easy to prepare and eating pancakes is a great way to start your day. Beat and mix Coconut milk, two eggs and almond extract together in a medium-sized bowl. In a separate bowl, mix salt, baking powder, sugar, flour and grated coconut. Blend the dry and wet mixtures together until it is moistened. Cut banana into several bits and slices place in batter. If you want to have thinner pancakes, simply add more coconut milk. Heat an ample amount of coconut oil into a frying pan. Place batter into the pan when it is hot enough. Cook until small bubbles arise. Flip and cook both sides until done.

Luscious Coco-Chicken Soup

Ingredients:

2 cans of Coconut Milk
2 tablespoons of Virgin Coconut Oil
Sea salt and pepper
1 chopped onion
2 sliced carrots
Chopped cauliflower (desired amount)
2 sticks of celery
½ cup of peas
9 ounces of chopped chicken
1 cup of water

Procedure:

Preparing soup is quick and easy and is perfect for cold seasons. Simply sauté the vegetables and chicken pieces in coconut oil until chicken turns golden brown. Mix it with Coconut Milk, water and seasonings. Leave it to simmer for 30 minutes then serve it warm

Basic Oven Omelets

Ingredients:

2 Eggs
2 tablespoons of Virgin Coconut Oil
Salt and Pepper

Procedure:

Preheat oven to 400 degrees Fahrenheit or 200 degrees Celsius. Warm up the baking dish with Coconut Oil until it is hot. Remove from oven, put the egg mixture and bake it for 15 minutes. You will notice that it cooks when it starts to rise and develop volume several times increasing into slightly fluffy omelets. You can serve it as is or you can make it a little more special by topping it with your favorite ingredient.

Carrot Cake

Ingredients:

1cup of grated carrots
1 cup grams of brown sugar
¼ cup chopped walnuts
2 eggs
1 grated zest of orange
1 teaspoon of bicarbonate soda
1 teaspoon of ground cinnamon
1 teaspoon of liquid Virgin Coconut Oil
½ cup plain whole wheat flour

Procedure:

All you have to do to is to mix all the above ingredients together and put it in a baling tin lubricated with virgin coconut oil. Preheat oven at 180 degrees Celsius or 350 degrees Fahrenheit and let it bake for 40-60 minutes.

In Closing

Being healthy is all about smart choices. The small things that we use every day and the choices we make on a daily basis can actually matter a great deal to our overall health and wellness. In keeping ourselves and our loved ones healthy, choosing organic and natural substances is highly recommended. One such thing is Coconut oil, which as you may know by now is a 100% natural plant extract that has been studied by scientists and has been found to have components that provide wonderful health benefits. This eBook aimed to provide you with relevant information regarding all the aspects of your life in which coconut oil can help. I only hope that you use the knowledge you gained from reading this book in making healthy choices and improving your health.

Thank You For Purchasing The Book

Thank you for purchasing this book. I hope you enjoyed it and now have strategies you can implement to improve your health with coconut oil. I am hoping that you take action and become an active participant in re-establishing and then maintaining your health.

If you liked what you read you might want to head over to http://joshuacollinshealth.com and take a look at the other books authored by Joshua Collins.

Yours in Health,

Joshua

Other Health Related Books By Joshua Collins

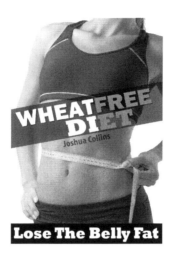

The Wheat Free Diet Book is available at
http://joshuacollinshealth.com/wheatfree

Wheat has been identified as a possible root cause of many chronic and debilitating medical conditions such as Celiac disease, diabetes and obesity. Don't become another statistic. This book can change your life!

Joshua Collins provides everything you ever wanted and needed to know about a Wheat Free eating program. He has also included some awesome recipes that are both nutritious and delicious and can easily be incorporated into your lifestyle. So if you are **"sick and tired"** of being **"sick and tired"** this book by Joshua Collins will benefit you.

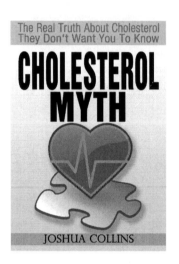

The Cholesterol Myth is available at http://joshuacollinshealth.com/

Joshua Collins, an expert in health and nutrition wrote this book to expose the truth about Cholesterol and to let you know what you can do to improve your heart health and overall health. He has done so in a concise, easy to understand way and produced this "fluff-free" book.

Medical Disclaimer

This book is intended as a reference guide only and not as a medical manual or medical advice. The sources and information provided in this book are strictly designed to assist you in making informed decisions regarding your overall conditions or problems. Please seek the advice of a qualified medical professional when it comes to making medical decisions, changing diets or exercise programs. This book, nor the information herein, is intended to replace or substitute any diagnosis, treatment or medication that has been prescribed or recommended by a health care provider, your doctor or a pharmacist. I strongly suggest you check with your medical care provider, pharmacist or doctor and follow their guidelines to create a well-balanced, nutritional diet and before beginning any new exercise, diet program or health related regime. Each person has different needs and requirements, based on their overall health situation. Please consult your physician before starting any new health programs.

9124548R00035

Printed in Great Britain
by Amazon.co.uk, Ltd.,
Marston Gate.